THE DHEA

Age Gracefully: How DHEA Supplements
Can Turn Back the Clock + The Proof, The
Myths, And The Answers

DR. BRIALLEN GERFRIED

Table of Contents

Introductory

DHEA (Dehydroepiandrosterone) is a steroid hormone that is predominantly produced by the adrenal glands, with smaller amounts occurring in the brain and gonads (ovaries and testes). It functions as a precursor to the sex hormones testosterone and estrogen, which are produced by both males and females. The following are several critical factors regarding DHEA:

1. Function: DHEA is a component of the synthesis of androgens and estrogens, which are the sex hormones for males and females, respectively. It is involved in a variety of physiological functions, such as energy levels, immune response, and overall mood.

2. DHEA Levels and Aging: DHEA levels reach their maximum during early adulthood and decrease as we age. When individuals reach their 70s and 80s, their DHEA levels are typically only 10-20% of what they were at their high point.

3. Health Consequences: Numerous health issues, including cognitive decline, decreased bone density, and impaired immune function, have been linked to low levels of DHEA. In contrast, certain studies indicate that the maintenance of healthy DHEA levels may enhance energy levels, improve mood, and support immune function.

4. Supplementation: DHEA supplements are occasionally employed to mitigate the effects of aging and to resolve a variety of health issues. Nevertheless, their utilization is contentious, and the scientific evidence that substantiates their advantages is inconsistent. The long-term safety and efficacy of DHEA supplementation are still being investigated, and it may interact with other medications and cause adverse effects.

5. Usage and Regulation: In certain countries, DHEA is available as an over-the-counter dietary supplement, whereas in others, a prescription may be necessary. A healthcare provider should superintend the use of the product to guarantee its safety and appropriateness.

It is ongoing research to comprehend the effects of DHEA on the body, and individuals who are contemplating DHEA supplementation should consult with their healthcare provider to discuss the potential benefits and risks.

CHAPTER ONE
Natural Production Of DHEA

The adrenal glands, which are situated on top of the kidneys, are the primary source of DHEA (Dehydroepiandrosterone) production in the human body. Furthermore, the brain and the gonads (ovaries in women and testes in males) produce smaller quantities. The following is a summary of the natural production process of DHEA:

1. Adrenal Glands: The adrenal glands are the primary source of DHEA production. Synthesis of DHEA from cholesterol occurs within the adrenal cortex through a sequence of enzymatic reactions. The process commences with the conversion of cholesterol to pregnenolone, which is subsequently converted to DHEA.

2. Steroid Hormone Pathway: DHEA functions as an intermediate in the steroid hormone biosynthesis pathway. It can be further converted into androgens (such as testosterone) and estrogens (such as estradiol) through additional enzymatic processes. This conversion takes place in a variety of tissues, such as the adrenal glands, gonads, and peripheral tissues.

3. Regulation: The hypothalamic-pituitary-adrenal (HPA) axis regulates the production of DHEA. Corticotropin-releasing hormone (CRH) is released by the hypothalamus, which activates the pituitary gland to secrete adrenocorticotropic hormone (ACTH). ACTH subsequently stimulates the adrenal glands to produce DHEA, cortisol, and other adrenal hormones.

4. Age-Related Decline: DHEA levels reach their maximum in early maturity and begin to decrease around the age of 30. DHEA levels are typically significantly lower than their optimum levels by the time individuals reach their 70s and 80s. This age-related decrease in DHEA production is a typical aspect of the aging process.

5. Function in the Body: DHEA is essential for the production of sex hormones, which are essential for reproductive health, secondary sexual characteristics, and overall physical and mental well-being. It also plays a variety of other functions, such as influencing brain function, metabolism, and the immune system.

The comprehension of DHEA's function in the body and the potential implications of its decline with age is facilitated by an understanding of its natural production and regulation.

Forms Of DHEA Supplements

DHEA supplements are available in various forms to accommodate different preferences and needs. The most common forms of DHEA supplements include:

Capsules/Tablets:

• **Capsules**: These are typically gelatin or vegetable-based and contain powdered DHEA. They are easy to swallow and come in various dosages.

• **Tablets**: These are compressed forms of powdered DHEA and also come in various dosages. They might be flavored or coated to make them easier to ingest.

Softgels:

• Softgels contain DHEA in a liquid form encased in a gelatin or vegetarian shell. They are easy to swallow and may be absorbed more quickly than tablets or capsules.

Sublingual Tablets:

• These tablets are designed to dissolve under the tongue, allowing for direct absorption into the bloodstream. This method bypasses the digestive system, potentially allowing for faster and more efficient absorption.

Creams/Gels:

• Topical DHEA creams or gels are applied directly to the skin. They are absorbed through the skin and into the bloodstream, offering an alternative for those who prefer not to take oral supplements or who may have difficulty with digestion.

Liquid Drops:

• DHEA in liquid form can be taken orally using a dropper. This form allows for flexible dosing and is absorbed quickly. It is also a good option for individuals who have trouble swallowing pills.

Micronized DHEA:

• Micronized DHEA refers to DHEA that has been processed into very fine particles to enhance its absorption and bioavailability. It is available in capsule, tablet, and powder forms.

Powders:

• DHEA powders can be mixed with water, juice, or other beverages. This form provides dosing flexibility and can be a convenient option for those who prefer not to take pills.

When choosing a DHEA supplement, it's important to consider factors such as dosage, form, bioavailability, and personal preference. Consulting with a healthcare provider is recommended to determine the most appropriate form and dosage based on individual health needs and goals.

Sourcing And Manufacturing

The sourcing and manufacturing of DHEA supplements involve several steps to ensure product quality, safety, and efficacy. Here is an overview of the process:

Sourcing

Raw Materials:

• **Wild Yam and Soy**: The primary #sources for the raw materials used in DHEA production are wild yam (Dioscorea villosa) and soy. These plants contain compounds such as diosgenin, which can be chemically converted into DHEA in a laboratory setting.

• **Quality Control**: The raw materials are carefully selected and tested for purity, potency, and contamination. This ensures that the starting materials are of high quality and safe for further processing.

Synthetic Production:

• While natural sources are used to derive compounds that are precursors to DHEA, the actual DHEA used in supplements is typically synthesized in a laboratory. This ensures a consistent and controlled production process.

Manufacturing

Conversion Process:

• The compounds extracted from wild yam or soy are chemically converted into DHEA through a series of controlled chemical reactions. This synthetic process is done in a laboratory and is monitored to ensure that the final product is chemically identical to naturally occurring DHEA.

Purification:

• The synthesized DHEA undergoes purification processes to remove any impurities or byproducts from the synthesis. This step is crucial to ensure the safety and efficacy of the final supplement.

Formulation:

• The purified DHEA is then formulated into various supplement forms, such as capsules, tablets, creams, gels, or liquids. This involves mixing the DHEA with other ingredients that aid in stability, absorption, and usability.

Quality Assurance and Testing:

Throughout the manufacturing process, rigorous quality assurance and testing protocols are followed. This includes:

• **Potency Testing**: Ensuring that each batch contains the correct amount of active DHEA.

• **Purity Testing**: Checking for contaminants such as heavy metals, microbes, and other impurities.

- **Stability Testing**: Assessing how the product holds up over time under different conditions.

- **Bioavailability Testing**: Ensuring that the DHEA can be effectively absorbed and utilized by the body.

Good Manufacturing Practices (GMP):

• Manufacturers are required to follow Good Manufacturing Practices (GMP) to ensure product quality and safety. This includes maintaining clean facilities, using proper equipment, and adhering to standardized procedures for production and testing.

Packaging and Labeling:

• The final product is then packaged in a way that protects it from contamination and degradation. Proper labeling is also crucial to provide consumers with information on dosage, usage instructions, ingredients, and any potential allergens or warnings.

Regulatory Compliance

FDA and Other Regulatory Bodies: In the United States, DHEA supplements are regulated by the FDA as dietary supplements. Manufacturers must comply with FDA regulations, including accurate labeling and ensuring that the product is safe for consumption. Similar regulatory bodies exist in other countries, each with their own set of guidelines and requirements.

Distribution:

• The finished DHEA supplements are distributed to retailers, pharmacies, and online marketplaces. From there, they become available to consumers.

By following these detailed steps in sourcing and manufacturing, companies aim to produce high-quality DHEA supplements that are safe and effective for consumers.

CHAPTER TWO
DHEA Vs. Other Hormone Supplements

DHEA (Dehydroepiandrosterone) differs from other hormone supplements in several ways, including its source, function, and applications. Here's a comparison between DHEA and some commonly used hormone supplements:

DHEA vs. Testosterone
Source and Function:

• **DHEA**: Produced primarily by the adrenal glands, DHEA serves as a precursor to testosterone and estrogen. It has a broader role in the body, influencing immune function, metabolism, and energy levels.

• **Testosterone**: Produced mainly in the testes in men and in smaller amounts in the ovaries in women, testosterone is a primary male sex hormone responsible for the development of male secondary sexual characteristics, muscle mass, and libido.

Uses:

• **DHEA**: Often used to counteract aging effects, support adrenal function, and enhance overall well-being. It can indirectly increase testosterone and estrogen levels.

• **Testosterone**: Used in hormone replacement therapy (HRT) for men with low testosterone levels, aiming to restore libido, muscle mass, and energy levels.

Administration:

• **DHEA**: Available in various forms including oral capsules, tablets, creams, and gels.

• **Testosterone**: Administered through injections, transdermal patches, gels, and implants.

DHEA vs. Estrogen

Source and Function:

• **DHEA**: As a precursor to estrogen, DHEA helps maintain overall hormonal balance and supports various bodily functions.

• **Estrogen**: Produced mainly in the ovaries, estrogen is the primary female sex hormone responsible for regulating the menstrual cycle, reproductive system, and secondary sexual characteristics.

Uses:

• **DHEA**: Used for general hormonal support, especially in aging individuals to boost overall hormone levels.

• **Estrogen**: Used in HRT for menopausal women to alleviate symptoms such as hot flashes, vaginal dryness, and bone density loss.

Administration:

• **DHEA**: Taken orally or topically.

• **Estrogen**: Available as oral tablets, transdermal patches, topical gels, and vaginal creams or rings.

DHEA vs. Progesterone
Source and Function:

• **DHEA**: Precursor to sex hormones, including progesterone.

• **Progesterone**: Produced in the ovaries after ovulation, it plays a critical role in regulating the menstrual cycle and maintaining pregnancy.

Uses:

• **DHEA**: Supports overall hormonal balance and well-being.

- **Progesterone**: Used in HRT to balance estrogen levels in menopausal women and to support pregnancy in women with progesterone deficiencies.

Administration:

• **DHEA**: Oral or topical.

• **Progesterone**: Oral capsules, vaginal suppositories, creams, and injections.

DHEA vs. Human Growth Hormone (HGH)

Source and Function:

• **DHEA**: Produced by the adrenal glands, influences the production of sex hormones.

• **HGH**: Produced by the pituitary gland, HGH stimulates growth, cell reproduction, and regeneration.

Uses:

• **DHEA**: Supports adrenal function, hormonal balance, and overall vitality.

- **HGH**: Used to treat growth hormone deficiencies, improve muscle mass, reduce fat, and enhance recovery and overall vitality.

Administration:

- **DHEA**: Oral or topical.

- **HGH**: Typically administered through injections.

Key Differences And Considerations

Function and Role:

- DHEA serves as a precursor to other hormones and has a broader role in supporting various bodily functions.

- Other hormone supplements (like testosterone, estrogen, progesterone, and HGH) directly replace or supplement specific hormones that have distinct and targeted roles in the body.

Indications:

• DHEA is used for general hormonal support and anti-aging benefits.

• Specific hormone supplements are used for targeted hormone replacement therapy to address particular deficiencies or medical conditions.

Regulation and Supervision:

• While DHEA is often available over-the-counter, other hormone supplements typically require a prescription and medical supervision due to their potent effects and potential side effects.

Choosing between DHEA and other hormone supplements should be based on individual health needs, hormonal levels, and medical advice. It's essential to consult with a healthcare provider to determine the most appropriate and effective treatment.

Legal And Regulatory Aspects

The legal and regulatory aspects of DHEA and other hormone supplements vary by country and are influenced by factors such as their classification, safety profiles, and intended use. Here is an overview of these aspects:

United States

DHEA:

• **Regulation**: DHEA is classified as a dietary supplement under the Dietary Supplement Health and Education Act of 1994 (DSHEA). As such, it is regulated by the Food and Drug Administration (FDA).

• **Availability**: Available over-the-counter without a prescription.

• **Requirements**: Manufacturers must ensure that DHEA supplements are safe, properly labeled, and do not contain misleading claims.

However, they are not required to prove safety and efficacy before marketing.

• **Quality Control**: The FDA monitors DHEA supplements post-market and can take action against products that are adulterated or misbranded.

Other Hormone Supplements (Testosterone, Estrogen, Progesterone, HGH):

• **Regulation**: Classified as prescription medications and regulated more strictly by the FDA.

• **Availability**: Require a prescription from a licensed healthcare provider.

• **Requirements**: Must undergo rigorous testing for safety and efficacy through clinical trials before receiving FDA approval. Manufacturers must adhere to Good Manufacturing Practices (GMP).

• **Monitoring**: The FDA monitors adverse events and can mandate additional warnings, restrictions, or product withdrawals if safety concerns arise.

European Union

DHEA:

• **Regulation**: Varies by country within the EU. Some countries classify DHEA as a prescription medication, while others allow it as a dietary supplement.

• **Availability**: In countries where DHEA is considered a supplement, it is available over-the-counter. In others, it requires a prescription.

• **Quality Control**: Subject to the regulations of the European Food Safety Authority (EFSA) or national regulatory bodies, which ensure product safety and proper labeling.

Other Hormone Supplements (Testosterone, Estrogen, Progesterone, HGH):

• **Regulation**: Treated as prescription medications and subject to stringent regulatory oversight by the European Medicines Agency (EMA) and national regulatory agencies.

• **Availability**: Only available with a prescription from a healthcare provider.

• **Requirements**: Must meet strict safety, efficacy, and quality standards before approval. Ongoing monitoring of adverse effects is required.

Canada

DHEA:

• **Regulation**: Classified as a natural health product (NHP) and regulated by Health Canada.

• **Availability**: Available over-the-counter but must meet specific regulatory requirements.

• **Requirements**: Manufacturers must obtain a product license and adhere to Good Manufacturing Practices (GMP). Products must be safe, properly labeled, and evidence-based claims are required.

Other Hormone Supplements (Testosterone, Estrogen, Progesterone, HGH):

• **Regulation**: Classified as prescription drugs and regulated by Health Canada.

• **Availability**: Require a prescription from a healthcare provider.

• **Requirements**: Must pass rigorous safety and efficacy evaluations before approval. Post-market surveillance ensures ongoing safety.

Australia

DHEA:

• **Regulation**: Considered a prescription-only medication and regulated by the Therapeutic Goods Administration (TGA).

- **Availability**: Only available with a prescription.

- **Requirements**: Subject to strict regulatory controls to ensure safety, quality, and efficacy.

Other Hormone Supplements (Testosterone, Estrogen, Progesterone, HGH):

- **Regulation**: Also regulated by the TGA as prescription medications.

- **Availability**: Require a prescription from a licensed healthcare provider.

- **Requirements**: Must comply with stringent safety and efficacy standards. Post-market monitoring and reporting of adverse events are mandatory.

General Considerations

Safety and Efficacy:

• **DHEA**: While generally considered safe for short-term use, the long-term safety and efficacy of DHEA supplements are not well-established. Regulatory bodies emphasize the need for consumers to use these supplements under medical guidance.

• **Other Hormone Supplements**: Have well-documented safety and efficacy profiles through clinical trials and are closely monitored for adverse effects.

Labeling and Marketing:

• **DHEA**: Must be accurately labeled with ingredients, dosage, and health claims supported by evidence. Misleading or unsubstantiated claims are subject to regulatory action.

• **Other Hormone Supplements**: Require detailed prescribing information, including indications, contraindications, side effects, and usage guidelines.

Consumer Awareness:

• Consumers should be aware of the legal status and regulatory requirements of DHEA and other hormone supplements in their respective countries. Consulting healthcare providers before starting any hormone supplementation is crucial for safety and efficacy.

Understanding these legal and regulatory aspects ensures that consumers make informed decisions and use hormone supplements safely and effectively.

CHAPTER THREE
Health Benefits Of DHEA

DHEA (Dehydroepiandrosterone) is often touted for its potential health benefits, especially as a supplement for aging individuals. Research on DHEA is ongoing, and while some benefits are supported by evidence, others are more speculative. Here are some of the potential health benefits of DHEA:

1. Anti-Aging Effects:

• **Skin Health**: DHEA may improve skin hydration, thickness, and elasticity, potentially reducing the appearance of aging.

• **Energy and Vitality**: Some users report increased energy levels and overall vitality.

2. Bone Health:

• **Bone Density**: DHEA supplementation has been linked to increased bone density in older adults, which can help prevent osteoporosis and fractures.

3. Immune System Support:

Immune Function: DHEA has immunomodulatory effects, which may enhance immune function and reduce inflammation.

4. Cognitive Function:

Mental Clarity and Memory: Some studies suggest that DHEA may improve cognitive function, memory, and overall brain health, particularly in older adults.

5. Mood and Emotional Well-Being:

• **Depression and Anxiety**: DHEA may have antidepressant effects and help reduce symptoms of depression and anxiety. It is thought to influence mood by affecting levels of neurotransmitters in the brain.

6. Sexual Health:

• **Libido and Sexual Function**: DHEA can boost libido and improve sexual function in both men and women, potentially through its conversion to testosterone and estrogen.

• **Menopause Symptoms**: In women, DHEA may alleviate menopausal symptoms such as hot flashes and vaginal dryness by providing a source of estrogen.

7. Metabolic Health:

• **Weight Management**: DHEA might help with weight loss and management by influencing fat metabolism and reducing abdominal fat.

• **Insulin Sensitivity**: Some evidence suggests that DHEA can improve insulin sensitivity and reduce the risk of type 2 diabetes.

8. Cardiovascular Health:

• **Cholesterol Levels**: DHEA supplementation may help lower LDL ("bad") cholesterol and increase HDL ("good") cholesterol, potentially reducing the risk of cardiovascular diseases.

• **Blood Pressure**: There is some evidence that DHEA can help lower blood pressure, contributing to overall heart health.

9. Hormonal Balance:

• **Adrenal Insufficiency**: For individuals with adrenal insufficiency, DHEA supplementation can help restore hormonal balance and alleviate symptoms of fatigue and weakness.

• **Androgen Deficiency**: DHEA can be beneficial in conditions where androgen levels are low, helping to restore normal hormonal function.

Considerations And Precautions

Individual Variability:

• The effects of DHEA can vary widely among individuals. What works for one person may not work for another, and some may experience side effects.

Potential Side Effects:

• Side effects can include acne, hair loss, increased facial hair in women, mood changes, and potential impacts on hormone-sensitive conditions (like breast cancer or prostate cancer).

Dosage and Monitoring:

• It is crucial to use DHEA under the guidance of a healthcare provider to determine the appropriate dosage and monitor for any adverse effects. Blood levels of DHEA and other hormones should be checked periodically.

Long-term Safety:

• The long-term safety of DHEA supplementation is not well-established. Ongoing research is needed to fully understand the potential risks and benefits.

DHEA supplementation offers various potential health benefits, particularly in the context of aging and hormonal imbalances. However, its use should be approached with caution, and it is essential to consult with a healthcare provider to ensure safe and effective use.

DHEA And Disease Prevention

DHEA (Dehydroepiandrosterone) has been studied for its potential role in disease prevention. While research is ongoing and not all claims are conclusively proven, there are several areas where DHEA may contribute to reducing the risk or severity of certain diseases:

1. Cardiovascular Disease

Potential Benefits:

Cholesterol Levels: DHEA may help improve lipid profiles by lowering LDL ("bad") cholesterol and increasing HDL ("good") cholesterol.

Blood Pressure: Some studies suggest DHEA can help lower blood pressure, which is a significant risk factor for heart disease.

Mechanism:

• The potential cardioprotective effects may be due to DHEA's role in reducing inflammation, improving endothelial function, and influencing lipid metabolism.

2. Osteoporosis

Potential Benefits:

• **Bone Density**: DHEA supplementation has been shown to increase bone mineral density, particularly in postmenopausal women and older men, which helps prevent osteoporosis and fractures.

Mechanism:

• DHEA acts as a precursor to estrogen and testosterone, both of which are critical for maintaining bone density.

3. Diabetes and Metabolic Syndrome

Potential Benefits:

• **Insulin Sensitivity**: DHEA may improve insulin sensitivity, helping to regulate blood sugar levels.

• **Weight Management**: It can influence fat metabolism, potentially aiding in weight management and reducing abdominal fat, which is a risk factor for metabolic syndrome and type 2 diabetes.

Mechanism:

• The hormone's role in modulating glucose metabolism and reducing inflammation may contribute to its beneficial effects on metabolic health.

4. Cognitive Decline and Neurodegenerative Diseases

Potential Benefits:

• **Cognitive Function**: DHEA has been associated with improved memory and cognitive function in some studies.

• **Neuroprotection**: There is evidence to suggest DHEA might have neuroprotective effects that could help in conditions like Alzheimer's disease.

Mechanism:

• DHEA may influence brain function through its effects on neurotransmitter levels, neurogenesis, and anti-inflammatory properties.

5. *Immune System Disorders*

Potential Benefits:

• **Immune Function**: DHEA has immunomodulatory effects that can enhance immune response and reduce inflammation.

Mechanism:

• By modulating the immune system, DHEA can potentially help prevent autoimmune diseases and infections.

6. Cancer

Potential Benefits:

• **Hormone-Sensitive Cancers**: There is some evidence suggesting that DHEA might have protective effects against certain types of cancers, such as breast and prostate cancer.

Mechanism:

• The hormone's influence on estrogen and testosterone levels might impact the development and progression of hormone-sensitive cancers. However, this is a double-edged sword, as inappropriate supplementation could also potentially promote cancer in susceptible individuals.

7. Mood Disorders and Depression

Potential Benefits:

• **Mood Enhancement**: DHEA has been found to have antidepressant effects and may help alleviate symptoms of depression and anxiety.

Mechanism:

• The mood-enhancing effects of DHEA are thought to be due to its impact on neurotransmitter synthesis and receptor sensitivity.

CHAPTER FOUR
Considerations And Precautions

Individual Variability:

• The effectiveness and safety of DHEA can vary widely among individuals, depending on their specific health status and hormonal balance.

Side Effects:

• Potential side effects include acne, hair loss, mood changes, and effects on hormone-sensitive tissues.

Medical Supervision:

• Due to the potential risks, DHEA supplementation should be done under medical supervision, with appropriate dosing and monitoring.

Long-term Safety:

• The long-term safety of DHEA supplementation is not fully established, and ongoing research is necessary to understand its benefits and risks better.

DHEA has potential benefits in disease prevention, particularly in areas related to cardiovascular health, bone density, metabolic health, cognitive function, immune support, cancer prevention, and mood disorders. However, its use should be approached cautiously, with proper medical guidance and consideration of individual health conditions.

Safety And Side Effects

DHEA (Dehydroepiandrosterone) supplementation, while generally considered safe for short-term use in appropriate doses, can have potential side effects and risks. Here's an overview of the safety considerations and possible side effects associated with DHEA:

Safety Considerations

Hormonal Effects:

• DHEA is a precursor to testosterone and estrogen. Supplementing with DHEA can lead to increased levels of these hormones, which may cause hormonal imbalances, especially in individuals with underlying conditions or hormone-sensitive cancers.

Interactions with Medications:

• DHEA can interact with various medications, including corticosteroids, insulin, and medications metabolized by the liver. It may affect their effectiveness or increase the risk of side effects. Consultation with a healthcare provider is essential if you are taking medications.

Long-term Use:

• The long-term safety of DHEA supplementation is not well-established. Prolonged use may lead to adverse effects, such as changes in lipid profiles, liver function, and cardiovascular health. Regular monitoring is recommended.

Adverse Effects in Certain Populations:

• People with hormone-sensitive conditions such as breast cancer, prostate cancer, endometriosis, and polycystic ovary syndrome (PCOS) should avoid DHEA supplementation or use it only under strict medical supervision due to potential exacerbation of their condition.

Quality of Supplements:

• The supplement industry is not tightly regulated, and the quality and purity of DHEA supplements can vary. Choose reputable brands that adhere to Good Manufacturing Practices (GMP) and third-party testing for quality assurance.

Potential Side Effects

Androgenic Effects:

• In women, DHEA supplementation can cause virilization symptoms, such as acne, increased facial hair growth (hirsutism), deepening of voice, and menstrual irregularities.

Mood Changes:

• DHEA may affect mood and behavior, causing irritability, agitation, or changes in emotional stability.

Cardiovascular Effects:

• Some studies suggest that DHEA might alter lipid profiles, potentially increasing LDL cholesterol levels and affecting cardiovascular health. This effect can vary among individuals.

Skin Reactions:

• Skin reactions, including acne and oily skin, are common side effects of DHEA supplementation, particularly at higher doses.

Other Potential Side Effects:

• Headaches, fatigue, insomnia, gastrointestinal upset, and dizziness have been reported in some individuals using DHEA supplements.

Precautions

Consultation with Healthcare Provider:

• Before starting DHEA supplementation, especially at higher doses or for extended periods, consult with a healthcare provider. They can assess your individual health status, discuss potential risks and benefits, and recommend appropriate dosages.

Monitoring:

• Regular monitoring of hormone levels, lipid profiles, liver function, and overall health is important when using DHEA supplements. Adjustments to dosage or discontinuation may be necessary based on monitoring results.

Dosage:

• Start with low doses of DHEA and gradually increase as tolerated. There is no established standard dose, as individual responses can vary widely.

Duration of Use:

• Use DHEA supplements for short-term purposes unless otherwise directed by a healthcare provider. Long-term use should be based on ongoing evaluation of benefits versus risks.

While DHEA supplementation may offer potential benefits in certain health conditions, it is crucial to approach its use with caution due to potential side effects and interactions. Consulting with a healthcare provider is essential to determine if DHEA supplementation is appropriate for you and to ensure safe and effective use.

CHAPTER FIVE
DHEA For Men

DHEA (Dehydroepiandrosterone) supplementation is sometimes used by men for various health benefits, particularly as they age and DHEA levels naturally decline. Here's an overview of how DHEA may affect men's health, potential benefits, considerations, and safety aspects:

Potential Benefits for Men

Testosterone Production:

• DHEA is a precursor to testosterone. Supplementing with DHEA may support testosterone production, potentially improving libido, muscle mass, and overall energy levels in men with low testosterone levels.

Bone Health:

• DHEA has been linked to increased bone mineral density, which is beneficial for maintaining bone strength and reducing the risk of osteoporosis, especially in older men.

Metabolic Health:

• DHEA may improve insulin sensitivity and glucose metabolism, which could be beneficial for men with insulin resistance or those at risk of developing type 2 diabetes.

Mood and Well-being:

• Some studies suggest that DHEA supplementation can improve mood, reduce symptoms of depression, and enhance overall psychological well-being in men.

Anti-aging Effects:

• DHEA is often marketed for its potential anti-aging effects, including improving skin health, enhancing cognitive function, and supporting overall vitality in aging men.

Considerations and Safety

Hormonal Effects:

• DHEA supplementation can increase levels of testosterone and estrogen. While this can be beneficial for men with low testosterone, it may also lead to hormonal imbalances or exacerbate hormone-sensitive conditions such as prostate cancer.

Individual Response:

• Responses to DHEA supplementation can vary widely among individuals. Some men may experience significant benefits, while others may not notice any changes or may experience side effects.

Side Effects:

• Common side effects of DHEA supplementation in men may include acne, oily skin, hair loss, mood changes, and gastrointestinal upset. Higher doses can increase the likelihood of adverse effects.

Interactions with Medications:

• DHEA can interact with medications such as corticosteroids, insulin, and medications metabolized by the liver. It's important to consult with a healthcare provider before starting DHEA supplementation, especially if you are taking medications.

Long-term Use:

• The long-term safety of DHEA supplementation is not well-established. Regular monitoring of hormone levels, liver function, and overall health is recommended if using DHEA long-term.

Dosage and Administration

• **Dosage**: There is no established standard dose for DHEA supplementation. It's advisable to start with a low dose (typically 25-50 mg per day) and adjust based on individual response and monitoring.

- **Form**: DHEA supplements are available in various forms, including capsules, tablets, creams, and gels. Choose a form that suits your preference and consider factors like absorption rate and convenience.

DHEA supplementation may offer potential benefits for men's health, particularly in supporting testosterone production, bone health, metabolic function, and overall well-being.

However, it should be used cautiously, under medical supervision, to minimize risks and ensure safe and effective use. Consulting with a healthcare provider is essential to determine if DHEA supplementation is appropriate for your individual health needs and to monitor for any potential side effects or interactions.

DHEA For Women

DHEA (Dehydroepiandrosterone) supplementation is sometimes used by women for various health benefits, particularly as they age and DHEA levels naturally decline. Here's an overview of how DHEA may affect women's health, potential benefits, considerations, and safety aspects:

Potential Benefits for Women

Hormonal Balance:

• DHEA is a precursor to both testosterone and estrogen. Supplementing with DHEA may help balance these hormones, potentially alleviating symptoms associated with hormone imbalances, such as irregular periods, low libido, and mood swings.

Bone Health:

• DHEA has been associated with increased bone mineral density, which is beneficial for maintaining bone strength and reducing the risk of osteoporosis, especially in postmenopausal women.

Libido and Sexual Function:

• DHEA supplementation may improve libido and sexual function in women, potentially enhancing overall sexual satisfaction and well-being.

Menopausal Symptoms:

• Some women use DHEA to alleviate symptoms of menopause, such as hot flashes, vaginal dryness, and mood swings. DHEA serves as a source of estrogen, which declines during menopause.

Cognitive Function:

• There is some evidence suggesting that DHEA may support cognitive function and memory, which can be beneficial for women experiencing cognitive decline with age.

Energy and Vitality:

• DHEA supplementation is sometimes used to boost energy levels and overall vitality, particularly in women feeling fatigued or experiencing reduced stamina.

Considerations and Safety

Hormonal Effects:

• DHEA supplementation can increase testosterone and estrogen levels. While this can be beneficial for balancing hormones, it may also lead to hormonal imbalances or exacerbate conditions like polycystic ovary syndrome (PCOS) or hormone-sensitive cancers.

Individual Response:

• Responses to DHEA supplementation can vary among women. Some may experience significant benefits, while others may not notice any changes or may experience side effects.

Side Effects:

• Common side effects of DHEA supplementation in women may include acne, oily skin, hair loss, menstrual irregularities, mood changes, and gastrointestinal upset.

Higher doses can increase the likelihood of adverse effects.

Interactions with Medications:

• DHEA can interact with medications such as hormone therapies, corticosteroids, insulin, and medications metabolized by the liver. It's important to consult with a healthcare provider before starting DHEA supplementation, especially if you are taking medications.

Long-term Use:

• The long-term safety of DHEA supplementation is not well-established. Regular monitoring of hormone levels, liver function, and overall health is recommended if using DHEA long-term.

Dosage and Administration

• **Dosage**: There is no established standard dose for DHEA supplementation. It's advisable to start with a low dose (typically 25-50 mg per day) and adjust based on individual response and monitoring.

• **Form**: DHEA supplements are available in various forms, including capsules, tablets, creams, and gels. Choose a form that suits your preference and consider factors like absorption rate and convenience.

DHEA supplementation may offer potential benefits for women's health, particularly in supporting hormonal balance, bone health, libido, menopausal symptoms, cognitive function, and overall vitality.

However, it should be used cautiously, under medical supervision, to minimize risks and ensure safe and effective use. Consulting with a healthcare provider is essential to determine if DHEA supplementation is appropriate for your individual health needs and to monitor for any potential side effects or interactions.

DHEA For Seniors

DHEA (Dehydroepiandrosterone) supplementation in seniors is a topic of interest due to its potential benefits in managing age-related hormonal changes and promoting overall health. Here's an overview of how DHEA may affect seniors, its potential benefits, considerations, and safety aspects:

Potential Benefits for Seniors

Hormonal Support:

• DHEA levels decline with age, and supplementation may help restore some of these hormone levels, potentially improving overall hormonal balance.

Bone Health:

• DHEA has been associated with increased bone mineral density, which is crucial for maintaining bone strength and reducing the risk of osteoporosis in seniors.

Muscle Mass and Strength:

• Some studies suggest that DHEA supplementation may help preserve muscle mass and strength in older adults, which is important for maintaining mobility and reducing frailty.

Cognitive Function:

• DHEA has been investigated for its potential role in supporting cognitive function and memory in seniors, although more research is needed to confirm its effectiveness.

Immune Function:

• DHEA has immunomodulatory effects that may support immune function in older adults, potentially reducing the risk of infections and enhancing overall health.

Energy and Vitality:

• Seniors may experience increased energy levels and improved overall vitality with DHEA supplementation, although individual responses can vary.

Considerations and Safety

Hormonal Effects:

• DHEA supplementation can affect hormone levels, including testosterone and estrogen. Seniors should use DHEA supplements under medical supervision to monitor for hormonal imbalances or exacerbation of existing health conditions.

Individual Response:

• Responses to DHEA supplementation can vary among seniors. It's essential to start with low doses and monitor for any adverse effects or improvements in health outcomes.

Side Effects:

• Common side effects of DHEA supplementation may include acne, oily skin, hair loss, mood changes, gastrointestinal upset, and in women, virilization symptoms such as increased facial hair growth.

Interactions with Medications:

• DHEA can interact with medications such as hormone therapies, corticosteroids, insulin, and medications metabolized by the liver. Seniors should consult with a healthcare provider before starting DHEA supplementation, especially if they are taking medications.

Long-term Use:

• The long-term safety of DHEA supplementation in seniors is not well-established. Regular monitoring of hormone levels, liver function, and overall health is recommended if using DHEA long-term.

Dosage and Administration

• **Dosage**: There is no established standard dose for DHEA supplementation. Seniors should start with a low dose (typically 25-50 mg per day) and adjust based on individual response and monitoring.

• **Form**: DHEA supplements are available in various forms, including capsules, tablets, creams, and gels. Choose a form that suits preferences and consider factors like absorption rate and convenience.

DHEA supplementation may offer potential benefits for seniors in supporting hormonal balance, bone health, muscle strength, cognitive function, immune function, and overall vitality.

However, it should be used cautiously, under medical supervision, to minimize risks and ensure safe and effective use. Consulting with a healthcare provider is essential to determine if DHEA supplementation is appropriate for individual health needs and to monitor for any potential side effects or interactions.

DHEA For Athletes

DHEA (Dehydroepiandrosterone) supplementation has garnered interest among athletes due to its potential effects on muscle growth, recovery, and overall performance. Here's an overview of how DHEA may affect athletes, its potential benefits, considerations, and safety aspects:

Potential Benefits for Athletes

Muscle Mass and Strength:

• DHEA is a precursor to testosterone, a hormone crucial for muscle growth and maintenance. Some studies suggest that DHEA supplementation may support muscle mass and strength gains in athletes, especially during resistance training.

Recovery:

• DHEA may aid in muscle recovery after intense exercise sessions, potentially reducing muscle soreness and improving overall recovery time.

Energy and Endurance:

• Athletes may experience increased energy levels and improved endurance with DHEA supplementation, which can be beneficial for prolonged or intense training sessions.

Fat Metabolism:

• DHEA has been studied for its potential effects on fat metabolism, promoting lean body mass and reducing body fat percentage, which is advantageous for athletes seeking optimal body composition.

Cognitive Function:

• There is some evidence suggesting that DHEA may support cognitive function and focus, which can benefit athletes during training and competition.

Considerations and Safety

Regulatory Status:

• DHEA is considered a banned substance by various sports organizations, including the World Anti-Doping Agency (WADA). Athletes should be aware of doping regulations and potential consequences before considering DHEA supplementation.

Hormonal Effects:

• DHEA supplementation can increase testosterone levels, which may provide benefits for muscle growth and performance. However, athletes should use DHEA under medical supervision to monitor for hormonal imbalances and potential side effects.

Individual Response:

• Responses to DHEA supplementation can vary among athletes. It's essential to start with low doses and monitor for any adverse effects or improvements in athletic performance.

Side Effects:

• Common side effects of DHEA supplementation may include acne, oily skin, hair loss, mood changes, and gastrointestinal upset. Higher doses can increase the likelihood of adverse effects.

Interactions with Medications:

• DHEA can interact with medications such as hormone therapies, corticosteroids, insulin, and medications metabolized by the liver. Athletes should consult with a healthcare provider before starting DHEA supplementation, especially if they are taking medications.

Long-term Use:

• The long-term safety of DHEA supplementation in athletes is not well-established. Regular monitoring of hormone levels, liver function, and overall health is recommended if using DHEA long-term.

Dosage and Administration:

• **Dosage**: There is no established standard dose for DHEA supplementation. Athletes should start with a low dose (typically 25-50 mg per day) and adjust based on individual response and monitoring.

- **Form**: DHEA supplements are available in various forms, including capsules, tablets, creams, and gels. Choose a form that suits preferences and consider factors like absorption rate and convenience.

DHEA supplementation may offer potential benefits for athletes in terms of muscle mass, strength, recovery, endurance, and cognitive function. However, it should be used cautiously, under medical supervision, to minimize risks and ensure compliance with anti-doping regulations. Athletes considering DHEA supplementation should consult with a healthcare provider to determine if it is appropriate for their individual needs and to monitor for any potential side effects or interactions.

CHAPTER SIX
Practical Considerations

When considering DHEA supplementation, especially in various contexts like general health, aging, athletic performance, or specific conditions, several practical considerations should be kept in mind to ensure safe and effective use:

1. Consultation with Healthcare Provider:

• **Individual Assessment**: Before starting DHEA supplementation, consult with a healthcare provider, especially if you have pre-existing medical conditions or are taking medications. A healthcare provider can assess your health status, discuss potential risks and benefits, and recommend appropriate dosages.

2. Quality of Supplements

• **Reputable Brands**: Choose DHEA supplements from reputable brands that adhere to Good Manufacturing Practices (GMP). Look for third-party testing certifications to ensure quality, purity, and accurate labeling.

3. Dosage and Administration

• **Starting with Low Doses**: Begin with a low dose of DHEA (typically 25-50 mg per day) and gradually increase as needed, based on individual response and healthcare provider recommendations.

• **Forms of DHEA**: Consider the form of DHEA that suits your preferences and needs (e.g., capsules, tablets, creams). Factors such as absorption rate and convenience should be taken into account.

4. Monitoring and Adjustments

• **Regular Monitoring**: Monitor your health status, hormone levels (if applicable), and any potential side effects while using DHEA supplements. Regular check-ups with your healthcare provider are essential, especially for long-term use.

• **Adjustments**: Adjust the dosage or discontinue supplementation if adverse effects occur or if there is no perceived benefit. Follow healthcare provider guidance on adjustments based on monitoring results.

5. Potential Interactions and Side Effects:

• **Interactions**: Be aware of potential interactions between DHEA supplements and medications you are taking, including hormone therapies, corticosteroids, insulin, and liver-metabolized medications.

• **Side Effects**: Common side effects of DHEA supplementation include acne, oily skin, hair loss, mood changes, and gastrointestinal upset. Higher doses may increase the likelihood of adverse effects.

6. Long-term Use and Safety:

• **Long-term Considerations**: The long-term safety of DHEA supplementation is not well-established. Use caution with prolonged use and ensure ongoing monitoring of health parameters.

• **Safety**: Consider your individual health profile, age, and any underlying conditions that may affect the safety and efficacy of DHEA supplementation. Always prioritize safety over potential benefits.

7. Compliance with Regulations:

• **Anti-Doping Regulations**: Athletes should be aware that DHEA is considered a banned substance by many sports organizations, including WADA (World Anti-Doping Agency). Ensure compliance with anti-doping regulations if you are an athlete or participate in competitive sports.

DHEA supplementation can potentially offer benefits in various health contexts, but it requires careful consideration of individual health status, dosage, quality of supplements, monitoring, and potential interactions. Consulting with a healthcare provider is crucial to ensure safe and effective use of DHEA supplements tailored to your specific needs and circumstances.

Personalizing Your DHEA Regimen

Personalizing a DHEA (Dehydroepiandrosterone) regimen involves considering individual health needs, goals, and potential risks. Here are steps to help personalize your DHEA supplementation regimen:

1. Assess Your Health Goals:

• **Identify Goals**: Determine why you are considering DHEA supplementation. Whether it's for hormonal balance, muscle strength, cognitive function, or other specific health benefits, clarifying your goals will guide your approach.

2. Consult with a Healthcare Provider

• **Health Evaluation**: Schedule a consultation with a healthcare provider, preferably one familiar with integrative or hormone-related therapies. Discuss your health history, current medications, and any conditions that may impact DHEA supplementation.

• **Lab Tests**: Consider requesting hormone level tests (e.g., testosterone, estrogen) to assess baseline levels and monitor changes over time.

3. Choose the Right Form and Dosage

• **Forms**: Select a DHEA supplement form that suits your preferences and absorption needs (e.g., capsules, tablets, creams). Discuss with your healthcare provider to determine the most suitable form.

• **Initial Dosage**: Start with a low dose (commonly 25-50 mg per day) and gradually increase based on your healthcare provider's recommendations and individual response.

4. Monitor and Adjust

• **Regular Monitoring**: Monitor your health and well-being while taking DHEA. Pay attention to any changes in mood, energy levels, skin condition, or other potential side effects.

• **Adjustment**: Based on monitoring results and consultation with your healthcare provider, adjust the dosage or consider discontinuing if necessary. Regularly review your regimen to ensure it aligns with your health goals.

5. Consider Potential Interactions and Side Effects:

• **Medication Interactions**: Be aware of potential interactions with medications you are taking, such as hormone therapies, corticosteroids, insulin, and liver-metabolized drugs. Discuss with your healthcare provider to minimize risks.

• **Side Effects**: Watch for common side effects like acne, oily skin, hair changes, and gastrointestinal discomfort. Report any adverse reactions to your healthcare provider promptly.

6. Long-term Use and Safety:

• **Safety Guidelines**: Follow safety guidelines for DHEA supplementation, including avoiding long-term use without medical supervision. Regularly review your regimen's safety and efficacy.

7. Lifestyle Support:

• **Healthy Lifestyle**: Support your DHEA regimen with a balanced diet, regular exercise, stress management, and adequate sleep. These lifestyle factors can complement the benefits of supplementation.

8. Reassess and Adjust Over Time:

• **Periodic Reviews**: Schedule periodic reviews with your healthcare provider to reassess your DHEA regimen's effectiveness, adjust dosages as needed, and address any new health considerations.

Personalizing your DHEA supplementation regimen involves careful consideration of your health goals, consultation with a healthcare provider, monitoring for potential side effects and interactions, and maintaining a balanced approach to support overall health. By following these steps, you can optimize the benefits of DHEA while minimizing risks, tailored to your individual needs and circumstances.

CHAPTER SEVEN
Controversies And Myths

DHEA (Dehydroepiandrosterone) supplementation has been surrounded by various controversies and myths over the years. Here are some of the key controversies and myths associated with DHEA:

Controversies

Regulatory Status and Legal Issues:

• DHEA is classified differently in various countries. In some places, it is available as an over-the-counter supplement, while in others, it may require a prescription or is banned altogether due to concerns about its hormonal effects and potential misuse in sports.

Hormonal Effects and Risks:

• One controversy surrounds the potential for DHEA to increase testosterone and estrogen levels. Critics argue that this could lead to hormonal imbalances, especially in individuals with hormone-sensitive conditions like breast or prostate cancer.

Long-term Safety:

- The long-term safety of DHEA supplementation is not well-established. Concerns exist regarding its impact on cardiovascular health, lipid profiles, and liver function over extended periods of use.

Effectiveness for Anti-aging:

• DHEA has been marketed for its potential anti-aging effects, but scientific evidence supporting its effectiveness in this regard is mixed. Some studies suggest benefits for skin health, cognitive function, and bone density, while others show minimal impact.

Myths:

Myth: DHEA is a Miracle Hormone:

• There is a misconception that DHEA is a panacea for various health issues, including aging-related conditions, cognitive decline, and sexual dysfunction. While it may offer benefits in certain contexts, it is not a cure-all.

Myth: DHEA Boosts Athletic Performance:

• While DHEA is sometimes used by athletes for its potential muscle-building effects, its use is controversial due to its classification as a banned substance in many sports organizations. Evidence supporting significant performance enhancement is lacking.

Myth: DHEA is Safe for Everyone:

• DHEA supplementation is not universally safe for everyone. It may interact with medications, exacerbate hormone-sensitive conditions, and cause adverse effects such as acne, mood changes, and gastrointestinal discomfort.

Myth: DHEA is Completely Natural and Without Side Effects:

• While DHEA is a naturally occurring hormone in the body, supplementing with high doses can lead to side effects such as oily skin, hair loss, and hormonal disruptions. It should be used cautiously and under medical supervision.

Addressing Controversies and Myths:

• **Evidence-based Approach**: Base decisions about DHEA supplementation on current scientific evidence and recommendations from healthcare providers.

• **Consultation with Healthcare Providers**: Seek guidance from healthcare providers who can assess individual health status, recommend appropriate dosages, and monitor for potential side effects or interactions.

• **Awareness of Regulations**: Understand the legal status of DHEA in your country or region, especially if you are an athlete or subject to anti-doping regulations.

• **Balanced Perspective**: Recognize that while DHEA may offer potential benefits in certain situations, it is not a substitute for healthy lifestyle habits and should be used judiciously.

While DHEA supplementation holds promise for certain health conditions, it is essential to approach it with awareness of controversies, myths, and potential risks. Making informed decisions and consulting with healthcare professionals are crucial steps in ensuring safe and effective use.

Frequently Asked Questions

Here are some frequently asked questions (FAQs) about DHEA (Dehydroepiandrosterone) supplementation, addressing common queries and concerns:

1. Is it healthy to take DHEA supplements?

• In general, the use of DHEA supplementation in appropriate doses is considered safe for short-term use. Nevertheless, the long-term safety of this medication is not yet well-established, and it may result in potential adverse effects such as hormonal imbalances, mood swings, acne, oily skin, and hair changes. It is recommended that individuals with hormone-sensitive conditions or those who are taking medications consult with a healthcare provider prior to using this product.

2. What are the potential adverse effects of DHEA?

• Common adverse effects of DHEA supplementation include acne, oily skin, hair loss, mood swings, gastrointestinal distress, and, in women, virilization symptoms (such as increased facial hair). The probability of adverse effects may be elevated by administering higher concentrations.

3. What is the recommended method of consuming DHEA supplements?

• DHEA supplements are accessible in a variety of formats, including capsules, tablets, and lotions. It is advisable to commence with a low dose (usually 25-50 mg per day) and subsequently modify the dosage in accordance with the individual's response and the recommendations of the healthcare provider. The form and timing of administration may differ depending on personal preference and absorption considerations.

4. Is it possible for DHEA supplements to interact with medications?

• Certainly, medications such as insulin, corticosteroids, hormone therapies, and liver-metabolized pharmaceuticals can interact with DHEA. It is imperative to disclose all medications you are currently taking to your healthcare provider prior to commencing DHEA supplementation in order to reduce the likelihood of interactions.

5. Is DHEA a lawful substance?

• The legal status of DHEA is subject to variation by country and region. It may be required to obtain a prescription or be regulated in certain regions due to concerns regarding its hormonal effects and potential misuse in sports, while it is available over-the-counter as a dietary supplement in others.

6. Is it advisable for athletes to consume DHEA supplements?

• Due to its classification as a prohibited substance by numerous sports organizations, including the World Anti-Doping Agency (WADA), athletes should exercise caution when supplementing with DHEA. Before contemplating DHEA supplementation, athletes should be cognizant of anti-doping regulations and potential repercussions.

7. Is it possible for DHEA to assist in weight loss?

• The role of DHEA in weight loss is not well-supported by evidence. Although certain studies indicate potential advantages in fat metabolism and body composition, the results are inconsistent, and additional research is required to determine its efficacy in weight management.

8. What is the maximum duration of DHEA supplement use?

• The optimal duration of DHEA supplementation is not well-defined. Due to the absence of conclusive evidence for prolonged use and potential long-term safety concerns, it is generally advised for short-term use under medical supervision.

Supplementing with DHEA may provide prospective advantages for particular health conditions, hormone balance, and aging-related issues. Nevertheless, it is imperative to exercise caution and seek medical advice to guarantee its safety and efficacy.

It is essential to consult with a healthcare provider in order to address individual health requirements, monitor for potential side effects or interactions, and make informed decisions about DHEA supplementation..

Acknowledgement

The information contained in this book regarding DHEA (Dehydroepiandrosterone) supplements is intended solely for educational purposes and is not intended to serve as medical advice. The content is derived from personal experiences, scientific data, and research; however, it should not be used as a substitute for professional medical consultation, diagnosis, or treatment.

It is imperative to consult with a qualified healthcare provider prior to initiating any new supplement regimen, including DHEA, to ascertain whether it is suitable for your unique health requirements and conditions. DHEA supplementation may interact with medications, medical conditions, or other supplements that you are currently taking. It is imperative to obtain personalized guidance from a healthcare professional who is knowledgeable about your medical history and can offer customized recommendations.

The author, publisher, and distributors of this book are not liable for any negative repercussions, consequences, or damages that may arise from the use or misuse of the information contained within. Any information contained in this book is solely at your own peril. In order to guarantee the safe and effective use of DHEA supplements, the reader is advised to engage in additional research and consult with healthcare providers.

The results and benefits of utilizing DHEA supplements as described in this book are not guaranteed. The efficacy of DHEA supplementation may differ depending on a variety of factors, such as age, health status, and other individual disparities, and individual results may vary.

This disclaimer is acknowledged and agreed to by the use of this book, and you assume entire responsibility for your health and well-being.

Conclusion

Dehydroepiandrosterone (DHEA) supplementation is a subject of ongoing research and discussion, with the potential to provide benefits for hormone balance, aging-related concerns, and specific health conditions.

In conclusion, this is true. Nevertheless, it is imperative to approach DHEA supplementation with a meticulous examination of the individual's health status, objectives, and potential risks:

• **Benefits:** DHEA has the potential to support hormone homeostasis, bone health, libido, cognitive function, and muscle strength and recovery.

• **Safety:** Although short-term use in appropriate doses is generally regarded as secure, further research is necessary to investigate the potential side effects and long-term safety. Before utilizing this product, athletes, individuals with hormone-sensitive conditions, and those who are taking medications should exercise caution and consult with their healthcare providers.

• **Regulation:** The legal status of DHEA is subject to regional variation, with certain countries enforcing regulations in response to concerns regarding its hormonal effects and potential misuse in sports.

• **Personalization:** The process of personalizing a DHEA regimen entails consulting with healthcare providers to evaluate health requirements, monitor effects, and modify dosages as required.

• **Education:** Individuals can make more informed decisions about the use of DHEA supplementation by comprehending the controversies, misconceptions, and frequently asked questions that surround it.

Ultimately, it is essential to maintain a balanced approach and seek professional guidance in order to optimize benefits and minimize risks, despite the potential of DHEA supplements to achieve specific health objectives.

It is imperative to remain informed about the latest developments in DHEA supplementation in order to make well-informed decisions regarding personal health and wellness as research continues to develop.

About The Author

Dr. Briallen Gerfried's philosophy of medicine is deeply rooted in ethical responsibility, expertise, and empathy. She regards the practice of medicine as a sacred obligation to alleviate suffering and promote well-being, rather than merely a profession. A profound respect for the inherent dignity and value of each individual is the foundation of Dr. Gerfried's philosophy. She comprehends that each patient is distinctive, possessing their own set of experiences, beliefs, and obstacles.

In light of this, she endeavors to establish a compassionate relationship with each individual in her care by actively listening to their concerns and treating them with the uttermost respect and dignity. Dr. Gerfried is a proponent of holistic care, acknowledging that health is not merely the absence of disease, but a state of emotional, mental, and physical well-being.

She employs a comprehensive approach to diagnosis and treatment, taking into accounts not only the symptoms that are present but also the underlying causes and contributing factors. She endeavors to encourage her patients to participate actively in their own health journeys by fostering open communication and collaboration, directing them toward decisions that foster long-term vitality and resilience. Dr. Gerfried's practice is founded on the principle of ethical integrity. She is steadfast in her dedication to maintaining the utmost ethical standards in medicine, placing the welfare of her patients above all else.

She endeavors to act in the best interest of those entrusted to her care by meticulously evaluating the potential risks and benefits of each decision. Her interactions with patients, colleagues, and the broader healthcare community are driven by the unwavering principles of integrity, honesty, and transparency.

Dr. Gerfried's medical approach is fundamentally characterized by a commitment to ongoing learning and development.

She is profoundly dedicated to remaining informed about the most recent developments in medical research and technology, acknowledging the dynamic nature of healthcare and the significance of adapting to changing knowledge and practices.

She guarantees that her patients receive the most up-to-date, evidence-based care by adopting a lifelong learning perspective. A medical doctor is not merely a profession for Dr. Gerfried; it is a vocation to serve others with integrity and dedication.

She is committed to maintaining the utmost ethical standards in her practice, consistently prioritizing the welfare of her patients. In essence, Dr. Briallen Gerfried's philosophy as a medical specialist from Harvard University is defined by a combination of empathy, expertise, and a dedication to providing exceptional patient care.

THE END